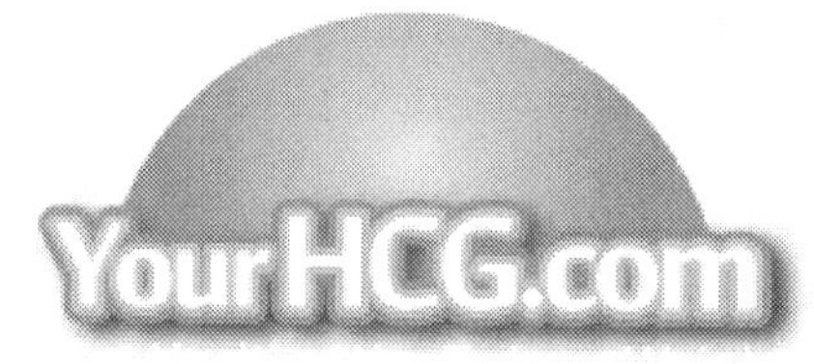

HCG Diet Recipes and Tips

To read more on the entire HCG diet, please visit www.YourHCG.com.

You can order a hard copy of this book from Amazon.com.

About Your HCG

YourHCG.com utilizes the highest standards to compliance protocols as well as manufacturing Kosher and Organic products. In addition, they provide homeopathic remedies that are made with individual care using traditional methods complying with current Good Manufacturing Practices (GMP). We implement high quality standards for the manufacturing of the remedies in strict accordance with the Food and Drug Administration (FDA) and the Homeopathic Pharmacopoeia of the United States (HPUS). Optimal reliability and reproducibility of the dilutions is guaranteed by the standardization of the manufacturing processes. Utilizing a time tested process; we rely on over 20 years of experience in the nutritional supplements to produce top quality products

Table of Contents

VLCD Diet Protocol

Maintenance Protocol

Dedication

Being overweight hurts more than just your physical appearance. It is linked to emotional issues, health issues and much more. This book is dedicated to anyone on the HCG diet who needs a little more variety in their foods. Oftentimes HCG dieters can find themselves being bored with the foods they can have. In this book, you will find over 100 recipes and tips to help you. You will love the delicious recipes. Here's to a healthy life.

-Your HCG

Breakfast:

- Black Coffee or
- Green Tea or
- Yerba Mate Tea or
- Wu Long Tea or
- Chamomile Tea

You may have as much as you desire. You may sweeten the tea and coffee with Stevia, but no other sweeteners should be used. Make sure that the Stevia doesn't contain any additional ingredients i.e. erythritol, dextrose, etc.

Lunch:

1. 100 grams (weighed raw) of grilled (no oil or fat) one of the meat choices below:

- Beef – This is not an ideal choice of protein. If you do have beef, limit it to a lean cut like Round Roast or London Broil and only have beef 2-3 times per week.
- Veal
- Fresh white fish (should not be frozen) – Ayr, Cat Fish, Cod, Coley, Dover Sole, Flounder, Flying Fish, Haddock, Hake, Halibut, Hoki, John Dory, Kalabasu, Lemon Sole, Ling, Monk Fish, Parrot Fish, Plaice, Pollack, Pomfret, Red & Grey Mullet, Red Fish, Red Snapper, Rohu, Sea Bass, Sea Bream, Shark, Skate, Tilapia, Turbot, and Whiting. ** The

best place to buy FRESH fish would be a local health food store if you live in a land-locked state.

- Chicken breast
- Shell fish (shrimp, crab, prawn, lobster, etc)
- Very occasionally we allow egg – boiled, poached or raw – to people who develop an aversion to meat, but in this case they must add the white of three eggs to the one they eat whole.

** (Per Pounds and Inches, American beef has almost double the caloric value of South Italian beef, which is not marbled with fat. The marbling is impossible to remove. In America, therefore, low-grade veal should be used for one meal and fish (excluding all those species such as herring, mackerel, tuna, salmon, eel, etc., which have a high fat content, and all dried smoked or pickled fish), chicken breast, lobster, crawfish, prawns, shrimps, crabmeat or kidneys for the other meal.)

2. One cup of one of the following vegetables:

- Spinach
- Chard
- Chicory
- Beet greens
- Lettuce of any kind
- Tomatoes
- Celery
- Fennel
- White, yellow or red onions
- Red radishes
- Cucumbers

- Asparagus
- Cabbage

These can be eaten raw, steamed, grilled or boiled. Do not mix vegetables in the same meal.

3. One of the following fruits:

- 1 apple
- 1 orange
- 1/2 grapefruit
- 1 cup of strawberries

4. One grissini breadstick or one Melba toast.

Dinner:

The same 4 choices as lunch.

Drinks Allowed:

Plain spring water, still mineral water, tea, coffee, Zevia. You should drink at least 2 liters of these liquids per day. We actually recommend drinking 1/2 of your weight in ounces per day. For example, if you weigh 200lbs you'll want to drink a min. of 100oz of water daily.
** Zevia is not on the original protocol. Use at your own risk.

Seasonings Allowed:

Salt, pepper, vinegar, mustard powder, garlic, basil, parsley, thyme, marjoram, etc. Spices should be in their natural form for best results. Watch for sugar, artificial sweeteners, mixed veggies, or foods not allowed on the diet (i.e. carrots) in your spices!

Misc...

- You may eat the breadstick and fruit as a snack in between meals instead of with your meals if you choose.
- No over the counter non-prescription drugs should be taken (with the exception of Aspirin). ** Consult your physician before discontinuing any medications, prescription or non-prescription.
- No cosmetics other than lipstick, eyebrow pencil and facial powder should be used.
- No creams, lotions or moisturizers that contain fat should be used. (Check the ingredient list. It is not safe to use if it contains "oil" or anything ending in "-ose")
- Those not uncommon patients who feel that even so little food is too much for them, can omit anything they wish (page 31 in Pounds and Inches)
- Massages are not recommended while on the HCG diet (page 42 in Pounds and Inches)

It is encouraged, but not required to do the following:

- Walk for one hour per day.
- Listen to stress reducing CDs.

- Do yoga as often as possible.
- Sweat for 20 minutes in a sauna as often as possible.
- Get twenty minutes of sun daily.
- Do not drink very cold beverages.

Beverages (10)

STRAWBERRY MARGARITA (minus tequila)

Cup of strawberries
Juice of ½ lemon
1 ½ packet Sweetleaf
4-5 ice cubes

Slice strawberries into chunks so they get down into the blender blades. Add a healthy squeeze of lemon juice. Add the Sweetleaf and blend until good and smooth. Add in ice cubes two at a time until your desired consistency... too much ice could make it watery so try it with 4-5 and then go from there. Pour into a tall glass and garnish with a fresh lemon wedge. You could also rim the glass with some lemon and a little Stevia for a little extra sweet/sour!
Serving Size - 1 Fruit, ½ Lemon

YUMMY VANILLA ICED COFFEE

Espresso strength coffee, cooled
1 Tablespoon milk
A few drops Vanilla Crème Stevia
Sprinkle of spice, if desired (cinnamon, pumpkin, etc)

Blend in blender with crushed ice until frothy. Delicious!!!
Serving Size - 1 Milk

BLOODY MARY

1 medium sized Tomato
Juice of half lemon
1 Teaspoon fresh cilantro, minced
Stevia to taste
1 clove minced garlic
¼ Teaspoon cumin
1/8 Teaspoon celery seed
Salt/pepper to taste
Tabasco to taste

Combine all ingredients in a blender and puree until reaches desired consistency. Serve chilled or over ice.
Serving Size - 1 Vegetable, ½ Lemon

VANILLA HOT COCOA

8 ounces hot water
5 drops Chocolate Stevia
2 drops Vanilla Creme Stevia

Place 8oz of water in a coffee mug. Add Stevia and mix.

CREAMY CAFE 'LATTE'

Pure coffee
1 Tablespoon of milk (only allowed 1 Tablespoon each day)
Vanilla Creme and Dark Chocolate Stevia drops

Place hot coffee in a coffee mug. Add Stevia and mix.
Serving Size - 1 Milk

PUMPKIN MOCHA WARM-UP
Coffee
1 Tablespoon milk
½ Teaspoon pumpkin pie spice (Check for sugars)
Dark chocolate or milk chocolate Stevia to taste

Place all ingredients in a blender and blend until frothy. Serve immediately.
Serving Size - 1 Milk

ORANGE DELIGHT
¾ cup crushed ice
1 orange
2 cups celery
5 drops Valencia Orange flavored Stevia

Mix in blender or juicer until smooth. Pour into glass and serve.
Serving Size - 1 Fruit, 1 Vegetable

SUMMERTIME LEMONADE
Water
Juice of lemon to taste (only allowed the juice of 1 lemon throughout the day)
Regular Stevia powder or drops to taste

Take 8 ounces of water and add the juice of ½ a lemon.
Add Stevia to taste
Serving Size - ½ Lemon

ORANGE DREAM

¾ Cup crushed ice
1 orange
**Removed the Orange Stevia drops
5 drops Vanilla Creme flavored Stevia

Mix in blender until smooth. Pour into glass and serve.
Serving Size - 1 Fruit

ENGLISH TOFFEE COFFEE

Pure coffee
English Toffee Stevia drops

Place coffee in a coffee mug. Add Stevia and serve.
Serving Size - 1 Milk

Fish and Seafood (18)

ASPARAGUS WITH GARLIC SHRIMP

100 grams small shrimp in their shells
Salt
Paprika, preferably Spanish
4 Tablespoons water
4 slices garlic cloves
¼ Teaspoon crushed red pepper flakes
Juice of 1 Lemon (split)
2 Tablespoon minced parsley
2 cups asparagus
Black pepper to taste

Shell the shrimp and sprinkle with salt and paprika. Heat the water, garlic and pepper flakes in a medium skillet. When the garlic is just beginning to brown, add the shrimp and cook, stirring, about 1 minute, or until just done and firm to the touch. Stir in 1 Tablespoon of lemon juice and parsley. In a separate frying pan, place asparagus with about ¼ inch of water in the bottom. Use the rest of the allotted lemon juice along with enough black pepper to taste. Cook on high until desired texture is reached. Serve immediately.
Serving Size - 1 Protein, 1 Vegetable

BOILED SHRIMP

100 grams shrimp
2-3 cups water (enough to cover shrimp in pan)
¼ cup apple cider vinegar
2 Tablespoons seafood seasoning

Add water, apple cider vinegar, seafood seasoning and shrimp to saucepan over medium-high heat. Let water come to a slow boil. When shrimp start floating, remove from heat and drain. Immediately place shrimp in ice water for 1 minute. Drain and serve immediately, or chill in refrigerator.
Serving Size - 1 protein

HOT WASABI WHITE FISH

100 grams whitefish
1 Tablespoon dry mustard
1 Tablespoon water
½ - 1 teaspoon wasabi powder (adjust to the desired level of spice)
½ Teaspoon ginger

In small dish, combine dry mustard, wasabi powder and 1 Tablespoon of water to make a paste. Add more water if needed. Mix in ginger. Add fish to dish and coat. Let stand for 15-30 minutes. Grill 4-5 minutes on the George Foreman until fish flakes. Or you can broil for 5-10 minutes depending on thickness of fish.
Serving Size - 1 protein

CRAB CAKES

100 grams crab meat
1 Grissini (ground into powder)
1 Teaspoon parsley
½ Teaspoon tarragon
½ Teaspoon paprika
½ Teaspoon lemon juice

¼ Teaspoon cayenne
¼ Teaspoon white pepper
¼ Teaspoon dry mustard
¼ Teaspoon seafood seasoning (optional)

Grind grissini into powder and place in a small dish. In a bowl, combine crab meat and remaining ingredients. Mix well and form into patties. Coat each side of patty w/ grissini powder. Brown in a non-stick skillet over medium heat for 3 minutes each side.
Serving Size - 1 Protein, 1 Breadstick

CURRIED BROILED FISH

100 grams fish
1 sliced tomato
½ lemon
½ - 1 Teaspoon curry seasoning

Preheat broiler. Place fish on broiler rack. Squeeze 1/2 lemon over fish. Sprinkle with curry seasoning. Place tomato slices on top of fish. Broil 8"-10" away from broiler for 10-15 minutes until tomato starts to blacken.
Serving Size - 1 Protein, 1 Vegetable, ½ lemon

NOW THAT'S GARLIC! SHRIMP

100 grams shrimp
4-6 cloves minced garlic
1/2 cup water
1/2 Teaspoon parsley
1/8 Teaspoon dried thyme
1/8 Teaspoon crushed red pepper
1 bay leaf

Heat nonstick pan over medium-high heat. Mix Tablespoon of water with red pepper, minced garlic, and bay leaf. Add to pan. Cook less than a minute. Be sure not to burn the garlic. Add shrimp. Cook 3 minutes. Remove shrimp from pan. Add the remainder of the 1/2 cup water, parsley, and thyme. Bring to a boil. Cook for 1-2 minutes until reduced by half. Return shrimp to pan & toss to coat. Discard bay leaf and serve.
Serving Size - 1 Protein

CREOLE FISH
100 grams whitefish
1 chopped tomato
½ cup water
1 - 2 Tablespoons Cajun seasoning

Preheat pan over medium-high heat. Cut fish into bite size pieces. Place fish in a sandwich bag. Add Cajun seasoning to coat. Pan fry coated fish in pan with water. Cook 3-4 minutes. If all the water cooks off, add more as needed. Add chopped tomato & stir-fry for another 5-10 minutes until tomatoes become tender and dish becomes soupy.
Serving Size - 1 Protein, 1 Vegetable

RED SNAPPER WITH FENNEL
100 grams red snapper (or any whitefish)
Fennel (weigh out your portion) - cut into 1" pieces
Juice of 1 lemon
2 Teaspoons fresh ginger
1 Teaspoon pepper

Place fish in shallow dish. Squeeze lemon juice in small bowl. Stir in ginger & pepper. Pour on fish and marinate in

refrigerator for 2 hours. Remove fish from marinade and place in glass baking dish. Place chopped fennel on top. Cover dish with lid or aluminum foil and bake @ 350 for 20-30 minutes or until fish flakes.
Serving Size - 1 Protein, 1 Vegetable, 1 Lemon

SPICY CILANTRO WHITEFISH

100 grams fish
Juice of 1/2 lemon
1/2 cup cilantro (pack measuring cup with cilantro leaves, not the stems)
3 cloves minced garlic
1 Tablespoon sambal oelek
1 Tablespoon water (as needed)
Red pepper flakes (optional)

Preheat oven to 400. In food processor, combine cilantro, garlic, and sambal oelek. Start to pulse and add water as necessary until reaches desired consistency. Place fish in baking dish or non-stick baking sheet. Squeeze on fresh lemon juice, then top with cilantro mix. Bake for 10-20 minutes, depending on thickness, until fish flakes. Top with red pepper flakes and serve.
Serving Size - 1 Protein, ½ Lemon

LEMON SHRIMP AND SPINACH

100 grams shrimp (peeled & deveined)
2 cups spinach
3 Tablespoons water
Juice of 1 lemon (or 1/2 lemon if you like things less lemony)
4-5 cloves minced garlic

Salt
Black pepper

Preheat non-stick skillet over medium heat. Add 3 Tablespoons water, garlic, and shrimp. Cook 5 minutes or until shrimp turns pink. Add water as necessary. Squeeze in juice of 1 lemon. Add spinach. Toss in salt & pepper. Cook uncovered until spinach wilts. Serve.
Serving Size - 1 Protein, 1 Vegetable, 1 Lemon

CAJUN SHRIMP KABOBS

100 grams shrimp
½ lemon
Fresh chopped parsley (to "chop" parsley, I simply use kitchen shears)

Place shrimp in bowl & add 1Tablespoon of Cajun Seasoning and toss to coat. Put shrimp on skewers (if using wood skewers, remember to soak in water for at least 20 minutes prior to use). You can also make kebobs with onion, tomato OR any other veggie allowed on protocol. Squeeze on lemon juice. Grill or broil until cooked through. Sprinkle with chopped parsley. Serve.
Serving Size - 1 Protein, ½ Lemon

SHRIMP STUFFED TOMATO

100 grams shrimp
1 tomato (allowed amount)
Juice of half lemon
1 Tablespoon parsley
Salt/pepper to taste
Tabasco (optional)

Place cooked shrimp in food processor. Pulse a few times to chop up shrimp. In a small bowl, combine chopped shrimp, parsley, lemon juice, salt and pepper. Cover and refrigerate for 30minutes - 1hour. When ready to serve, cut off top of tomato. Scoop out inside of tomato. Chop and combine inside of tomato with shrimp mix if desired. Fill tomato with shrimp mix. Top with a couple of dashes of Tabasco & serve.
Serving Size - 1 Protein, 1 Vegetable

CURRY SHRIMP
100 grams shrimp
Onion - chopped (allowed amount)
1 Teaspoon garlic paste (3-4 cloves minced)
1/8 cup water
½ Teaspoon curry powder
¼ Teaspoon cumin
Salt/pepper to taste

Preheat pan over medium heat. Add onion & garlic. Cook until translucent about 5-10 minutes. Add shrimp, seasonings and water. Mix & stir fry until cooked through. Serve.
Serving Size - 1 Protein, 1 Onion

ROCK LOBSTER WITH ASPARAGUS
1 Teaspoon salt
1 Teaspoon paprika
1/8 Teaspoon white pepper
1/8 Teaspoon garlic powder
2 Tablespoons water
Juice of 1 lemon - divided

2 - 10 ounces thawed rock lobster tails
** 3 ounces of lobster = 1 protein serving
2 cups asparagus
Pepper to taste

Split rock tails lengthwise with a large knife. Mix seasonings with lemon juice and water. Brush meat side of tail with marinade. Pre-heat grill and place rock tails meat side down and grill five to six minutes until well scored. Turn over lobster and cook another six minutes, brushing often with remaining marinade. Lobster is done when it is opaque and firm to the touch. Place asparagus in a pan with about ¼ inch water, juice from ½ lemon and pepper to taste. Cook on medium heat, and remove once the desired texture is reached.
Serving Size - 1 Protein, ½ Lemon

LEMON PEPPER FISH

100 grams white fish
Juice of ½ a lemon
1-3 cloves minced garlic
½ Teaspoon black pepper
¼ Teaspoon salt
¼ Teaspoon cumin powder
1/8 Teaspoon tumeric

Place fish in a small bowl. Then add garlic, black pepper, salt, cumin & tumeric. Ensure both sides are coated. Cover & marinate at least 1 hour in the fridge. Preheat oven to 400.
Place the fish in a non-stick baking dish and cover with the marinade. Bake 10-20 minutes depending on thickness, until fish easily flake. Squeeze with lemon juice & serve.
Serving Size - 1 Protein, ½ Lemon

LEMON OREGANO WHITE FISH WITH ASAPARGUS
100 grams white fish
Asparagus (allowed amount)
Juice of one lemon
1 Teaspoon oregano
Salt/pepper

Preheat oven to 400F. Snap off 'woody' ends of asparagus and discard. Tear off a large sheet of non-stick aluminum foil. In the center of this sheet, place asparagus spears and sprinkle with salt/pepper. Place white fish on top of asparagus. In small bowl, combine lemon juice & oregano, then pour over the fish. Fold up edges and completely seal packet on all sides. Bake 10-20 minutes, until fish flakes, serve.
Serving Size - 1 Protein, 1 Vegetable, 1 Lemon

Garlic Shrimp
100 grams shrimp
1 cup diced tomatoes or spinach
1/8 Teaspoon garlic
1/8 Teaspoon salt

1 cup water
Pepper to taste

Place in a saucepan and boil for 5 minutes or until shrimp is done.
Serving Size - 1 Protein, 1 Vegetable

YOURHCG.COM CIOPPINO

100 grams approved white fish
1 chopped tomato
2 cups water
2 -3 cloves minced garlic
1 Teaspoon parsley
¼ Teaspoon oregano
¼ Teaspoon basil
1/8 Teaspoon rosemary
1/8 Teaspoon fennel seeds
Salt/pepper to taste
Tabasco

Combine parsley, oregano, basil, rosemary and fennel seeds in food processor and grind. Add seasonings and all other ingredients except for fish & Tabasco to saucepan. Bring to a boil. Reduce heat, cover, and simmer for 30 minutes. Add fish and return to a boil. Reduce heat and cover and simmer for 5-15 minutes. Top with a few dashes of Tabasco just before serving.
Serving Size - 1 Protein, 1 Vegetable

Chicken (18)

BREADED CHICKEN TENDERS

100 grams chicken breast
1 Grissini (ground into powder)
½ cup water
¼ Teaspoon garlic powder
¼ Teaspoon paprika
¼ Teaspoon YourHCG.com Basic Seasoning (optional)
¼ Teaspoon cayenne (use less if you want them less spicy)
Salt/pepper to taste

Preheat pan over medium heat. In small dish, combine grissini powder, garlic powder, paprika, poultry seasoning, cayenne, and salt/pepper. (You could also use sandwich bag.) Add chicken to seasonings and fully coat. Add half of the water and chicken to pan. Cook for approx. 3-4 minutes each side depending on thickness of chicken. Keep adding more water as it cooks off. Serve immediately.
Serving Size - 1 Protein, 1 Breadstick

BAKED CAJUN CHICKEN

100 grams chicken breast
½ Tablespoon milk
½ Teaspoon Cajun seasoning

Preheat oven to 350. In a small dish, coat both sides of chicken with milk. Place chicken in glass baking dish. Sprinkle top with Cajun seasoning. Bake uncovered 20-30 minutes until chicken is no longer pink.
Serving Size - 1 Protein, ½ Milk

RED HOT CHILE CHICKEN

100 grams chicken breast
1 Tablespoon red chili paste
1 Tablespoon apple cider vinegar
3 cloves minced garlic
1 Teaspoon oregano
½ Teaspoon cumin
½ Teaspoon Stevia
Salt
Crushed red pepper (optional)

In sandwich bag, add all ingredients except chicken. Mix. Sprinkle chicken with salt and add the chicken to the bag. Seal and shake until coated. Place in fridge to marinate at least 1 hr. Cook chicken on George Foreman or under a broiler until done. Top with crushed red pepper and serve. Serving Size - 1 Protein

LEMON MUSTARD CHICKEN

100 grams chicken breast
Juice of 1/2 lemon
1 Tablespoon dry mustard
1/2 Teaspoon black pepper
1/2 Teaspoon oregano
1/4 Teaspoon cayenne pepper

Preheat broiler. Broil 1 side of chicken 5-10 minutes until slightly browned. In small bowl, add the rest of the ingredients and mix well. Spoon mixture onto chicken. Flip over and coat other side. Broil uncooked side 5-10 minutes or until no longer pink.

Serving Size - 1 Protein, ½ Lemon

KUNG PAO CHICKEN

100 grams chicken breast - cut into chunks
1 cup chopped onion
1-2 Teaspoon sambal oelek
Red pepper flakes (optional)

Marinade
1 part liquid aminos

Seasoning
Mash together in small bowl:
3 cloves minced garlic
1-2 teaspoons fresh minced ginger root

Sauce
Stir together in small bowl:
1/2 cup water
1-2 teaspoons liquid aminos

In small dish, combine marinade & chicken. Refrigerate 30 minutes - 1 hour. Preheat non-stick pan over medium-high heat. Cook chicken 5-7 minutes, browning on all sides. Add sambal oelek. Cook 1-3 additional minutes. Remove chicken from pan and set aside. Add onion to pan and cook until tender. Stir seasoning mixture in with onions. Cook 1-3 minutes. Add sauce mixture to pan. Cook 1-3 minutes. Re-add chicken to pan. Stir. Cook 1-3 minutes. Top with a few dashes of red pepper flakes (optional). Serve.
Serving Size - 1 Protein, 1 Vegetable

ORANGE GINGER CHICKEN

100 grams of chicken breast
2 cups cabbage cut in strips
1/4 cup water
Juice of ½ lemon
1 orange, peeled and squeeze the juice and add the pulp to sauce
½ Teaspoon for fresh ginger, slivered or grated
4 Tablespoons of Bragg's Liquid Aminos
Salt and pepper to taste

In a small bowl add all the ingredients except the chicken and cabbage. Whisk together. Place in a small frying pan and add chicken. Cook chicken until done remove chicken and add the cabbage with about ¼ cup of water. Cook cabbage until it's to your desired texture. Add chicken into pan. I had my cabbage cut long so it almost reminded me of lo mein.
Serving Size - 1 Protein, 1 Vegetable, 1 Fruit, ½ Lemon

SPICY FRIED CHICKEN

100 grams chicken breast
1 Tablespoon milk
1 Grissini breadstick
Sea salt
Pepper
Cayenne pepper to taste

Totally crush breadstick in food processor or put in a plastic bag and crush with a rolling pin. Dip chicken in milk and coat with the breadstick crumbs. Cook in a nonstick pan. Season with salt, pepper and cayenne. Serving Size - 1 Protein, 1 Milk, 1 Breadstick

SWEET N SPICY CHICKEN WRAPS

100 grams of chicken breast
4 cabbage leaves whole
1 small Gala apple, cored and chopped
2 Tablespoons of Braggs Liquid Amino Acids
Water
1 Tablespoon Tabasco
Course dry mustard
2 cloves of garlic minced
2 Tablespoons of water
Pepper to taste
1 Teaspoon garlic powder

In one small skillet put 100 grams of chicken in saute pan with 2 TBSP of Braggs Liquid Aminos, black pepper, and garlic powder. Cook chicken until done, adding water to deglaze pan and keep chicken moist. While chicken is cooking take another large pan (I use an 8" pan with high sides so the cabbage leaves lay open and will not tear) add water bring to a boil. Add cabbage leaves one at a time just to cook until cabbage leaf is tender and pliable. (I also remove the hard veins of larger leafs). As they are done take out and set to the side. Once the chicken is completely cooked remove chicken from the pan let cool and cut up...keep the juice from cooking chicken add the minced garlic 1 TBSP of mustard and about 2 TBSP of water. Bring to boil and cook your apples in this mixture. Once the apples start cooking down and tender, return the chopped chicken to the apples. Take your large steamed

cabbage leafs and spoon in the mixture and roll into wraps.
Serving Size - 1 Protein, 1 Fruit, 1 Vegetable

CABBAGE WRAPS
2-3 big cabbage leaves
1 cup shredded cabbage
** I removed the onion powder. To the purists, this would be considered mixing veggies.
1/8 Teaspoon garlic powder
1/8 Teaspoon Chinese Five Spice
1 piece Melba Toast
100 grams cooked chopped chicken breast or shrimp

Steam big cabbage leaves for 5 minutes. Move leaves over to side of steamer to make room for shredded cabbage. Steam both for 5 minutes. Remove shredded cabbage to a mixing bowl. Add chopped chicken or shrimp and spices. Mix and then wrap in big cabbage leaves. Garnish with Melba rounds.
Serving Size - 1 Protein, 1 Vegetable, 1 Melba toast

OVEN FRIED GARLIC CHICKEN
4 - 100 gram pieces of chicken breast
3 Teaspoons crushed garlic cloves
2 Tablespoon water
Dash of salt
Dash of pepper
½ Teaspoon oregano
½ Teaspoon basil

Put the garlic and water into the microwave for 25 seconds. Add salt, pepper and herbs to form a paste, adding more water if needed. Rub all over the chicken pieces. Lay the chicken pieces in a baking pan and bake on 425 for 30 minutes.
Serving Size - 1 Protein

SHISH KABOBS
100 grams chicken breast or shrimp
Choice of ONE - either onion or tomato
Juice of 1 lemon
¼ Teaspoon rosemary
¼ Teaspoon thyme
¼ Teaspoon cumin

Place chunks of meat choice and vegetable choice on a skewer. Season with herbs and lemon juice prior to grilling. Place on grill, rotating for 10 minutes
Serving Size - 1 Protein, 1 Vegetable, 1 Lemon

GARLIC CHICKEN
4 - 100 gram chicken breast (4 servings)
1 cup of diced onion
3-5 cloves garlic - unpeeled & left whole
Juice of half lemon
Black pepper to taste

Preheat oven to 350. Heat non-stick saucepan over medium. Add the onion. Stir constantly until tender, about 5-10 minutes. Transfer onions to glass baking dish. Place chicken atop onions. Squeeze on lemon juice & sprinkle with pepper. Place garlic around and on the chicken. Cover

tightly either with lid or aluminum foil. Cook for 30-45 minutes or until chicken is no longer pink.
Serving Size - 1 Protein, 1 Vegetable, ½ Lemon

BLACKENED CHICKEN SALAD

100 grams chicken breast
1 Teaspoon paprika
½ Teaspoon garlic powder
¼ Teaspoon oregano
¼ Teaspoon thyme
¼ Teaspoon white pepper
¼ Teaspoon black pepper
¼ Teaspoon ground red pepper
Spinach or salad greens (as allowed)

Combine all spices and rub on chicken. Grill until no longer pink. Serve over spinach or salad greens.
Serving Size - 1 Protein, 1 Vegetable

BONELESS HOT WINGS

100 grams chicken breast
¼ cup vinegar
¼ cup water
1-2 Tablespoons cayenne pepper
1-2 Tablespoons chili powder (adjust as needed)

In small bowl, mix vinegar, water, and cayenne pepper. Add chicken to marinade and refrigerate for 1-2 hrs. Preheat oven to 350. Add chili powder to a small dish and dip chicken in chili powder. Place on rack in baking pan. Bake 15-20 minutes turning halfway through.
Serving Size - 1 Protein

LEMON ROSEMARY CHICKEN

100 grams chicken breast
Juice of ½ a lemon
½ Teaspoon rosemary
¼ Teaspoon pepper
1-2 cloves minced garlic

Heat non-stick pan over medium-high heat. In small bowl, grate lemon peel. Add lemon juice, rosemary, pepper, and garlic. Toss in chicken. Place chicken in skillet. Cook 5 minutes brushing with remaining juice mixture. Turn over chicken and cook 5 more minutes or until juices run clear.
Serving Size - 1 Protein, ½ Lemon

MELBA DELIGHT

1 Melba toast
100 grams of chicken breast - sliced
1 slice tomato
Pinch of oregano
Pinch of salt

Cook chicken with salt and oregano. Serve with sliced tomatoes and Melba toast.
Serving Size - 1 Protein, 1 Vegetable, 1 Melba toast

Chicken & Tomatoes

100 grams of chicken breast
1 cup pureed tomato
1 cup water
½ Teaspoon sage
½ Teaspoon garlic powder
½ Teaspoon salt

½ teaspoon pepper

Place chicken in a baking dish. In a small bowl, mix water, sage, garlic, salt, and pepper. Pour sauce over chicken. Bake in the oven at 375 for 45 minutes.
Serving Size - 1 Protein, 1 Vegetable

Spicy Chicken
100 grams of chicken breast
¼ Teaspoon chili powder
¼ Teaspoon cayenne pepper
½ Teaspoon paprika
1 cup chopped tomatoes
2 Tablespoons apple cider vinegar
1 Tablespoon lemon juice
¼ Teaspoon garlic powder

Preheat oven to 350 degrees. Mix chili powder, cayenne pepper, and paprika in a small bowl. Spread liberally on both sides of chicken. Place in a small baking dish. In a separate bowl, add tomatoes, apple cider vinegar, and lemon juice and garlic powder. Mix well. Then pour over the chicken. Cook for 25-30 minutes at 350 degrees.
Serving Size - 1 Protein, 1 Vegetable

Beef (8)

BLUSTERY DAY CHILI

100 grams chopped London Broil or Round Roast
1 cup chopped tomatoes
½ cup water
2 cloves garlic crushed and minced
Pinch of garlic powder
¼ Teaspoon chili powder
Pinch of oregano
Cayenne pepper to taste (optional)
Salt and pepper to taste

Brown beef in small frying pan, add garlic. Stir in tomatoes and water. Add spices and simmer slowly until liquid is reduced.
Serving Size - 1 Protein, 1 Vegetable

MINI MEATLOAF

100 grams ground London Broil or round roast
½ teaspoon milk
1 Grissini breadstick, ground to powder
2-3 cloves minced garlic
½ Teaspoon dry mustard
¼ Teaspoon allspice
1/8 Teaspoon sage
Salt and pepper to taste

Preheat oven to 350. In small bowl, combine all ingredients and form into a small loaf. Place in glass dish, cover and bake 25-30 minutes. Uncover dish, and bake for 5-10 minutes. Serve immediately.

Serving Size - 1 Protein, 1 Breadstick, ½ Milk

HCG & FAMILY FRIENDLY ROAST

3 lb lean London broil or round roast, fat removed
6-8 large cloves garlic
1 Teaspoon dry oregano
1 Teaspoon sea salt
Fresh ground pepper
Water
1/6 head of cabbage OR 1 onion

Place the above in the roaster, add water until it is about 1 1/2 inches deep, and bake for 15 minutes on 350. Optionally, add potatoes and carrots for the family and cabbage or onion for the HCG dieter. Continue baking an additional 45-60 minutes depending upon how done you like your roast. Slice off 3 oz. of lean roast for the HCG dieter.
Serving Size - 1 Protein, 1 Vegetable

MEATBALLS

100 grams ground London broil or round roast
1 Grissini breadstick (ground into powder)
1 Tablespoon of milk
Pinch of parsley, basil, oregano, garlic, salt and pepper

Preheat oven to 425. In bowl, combine all ingredients. Then form into 1″ meatballs (makes about 6-7). Place in a baking dish on non stick aluminum foil and cook for 10 minutes, turning ½ way through.
Serving Size - 1 Protein, 1 Breadstick, 1 Milk

INSIDE OUT FRENCH DIP

100 grams sliced London broil or round roast
1onion - sliced into rings
1 cup water
2 cloves minced garlic
½ Teaspoon thyme
½ Teaspoon pepper

Preheat pan over medium heat. Add onions and garlic, cook for 5-10 minutes until tender. Add water, thyme and pepper. Reduce heat & simmer 5-10 minutes. Add steak and return to boil, then reduce heat and simmer for another 5-10 minutes. Serve steak & onions with au jus sauce.
Serving Size - 1 Protein, 1 Vegetable

MEAT IN TOMATO SAUCE

100 grams of any approved HCG meat
1 large tomato
¼ Teaspoon of garlic salt
¼ Teaspoon Italian Seasoning (make sure it has 0 carbs)

Slice up your tomato and put it into a sauce pan. Saute on medium for about 5 minutes. While they are being heated, occasionally smash the tomatoes with a spoon. While cooking the tomatoes, cook the meat you chose. When your tomatoes are heated and soft, they should have the consistency of THICK spaghetti sauce (or whatever consistency you prefer). After the meat is properly cooked, mix it together with the tomatoes. Add in your spices, stir.
Serving Size - 1 Protein, 1 Vegetable

ROSEMARY GARLIC STEAK

100 grams London broil or round roast
1 Tablespoon apple cider vinegar
1 Tablespoon rosemary
1 Teaspoon garlic paste (3-5 cloves minced)
½ Teaspoon crushed red pepper

In small dish, add vinegar and steak, then coat. In small bowl, combine rosemary, garlic and red pepper. Rub on both sides of steak. Place steak in small dish, cover and refrigerated for a minimum of 4 hours. Grill until desired doneness.
Serving Size - 1 Protein

YOURHCG.COM CINNAMON BEEF

100 grams of London Broil or Round Roast
Dash of cinnamon
Parsley flakes
Dash of black pepper
Dash of garlic powder

In a small bowl, add the cinnamon, parsley, black pepper and garlic powder in a bowl. Then take the 100 grams of beef and rub the seasoning all over. Then place on a George Foreman grill and cook to your liking. Serve with HCG friendly onion rings, cabbage, or a nice green salad.
Serving Size - 1 Protein

SOUTHERN STYLE GREENS

4 Tablespoons water
2 cups chopped beet greens
Dash of garlic salt
Red pepper flakes

Heat water on medium heat prior to boiling. Reduce heat; add greens and red pepper flakes. Saute a few minutes until tender. Sprinkle with garlic salt.
Serving Size - 1 Vegetable

SAUTEED GARLIC GREENS

6 cloves garlic, sliced
16 cups stemmed and roughly chopped chard
Squeeze of lemon
Red pepper flakes to taste
½ Teaspoon kosher salt

Heat garlic in large skillet over medium-low heat in a non-stick pan until garlic begins to turn golden, about 3 minutes. Transfer to a small bowl and set aside. Place greens, red pepper flakes and salt into skillet. Using tongs, turn greens until wilted enough to fit in pan. Raise heat to medium and cover. Cook 7-10 minutes, tossing frequently. Transfer greens to colander to drain. Return greens to pan and toss with reserved garlic. Squeeze with lemon just before serving. Refrigerate leftover greens in an airtight container for up to 3 days.
Serving Size - 1 Vegetable

SALSA

2 small tomatoes
Juice of ½ lemon
1/8 Teaspoon celery salt
1/8 Teaspoon chili powder
3 drops Clear Stevia
1 Teaspoon chopped fresh cilantro
1/8 Teaspoon garlic powder
1/8 cup Vinaigrette dressing (found under the "sauces tab)

Chop tomatoes. Combine dressing, lemon juice, spices and Stevia. Toss in tomato and refrigerate for at least 1 hour.
Serving Size - 1 Vegetable, ½ Lemon

GOOD FOR YOU ONION RINGS

1 cup sliced onions
1 Melba toast or Grissini breadstick
1 Tablespoon milk
¼ Teaspoon cayenne pepper
¼ Teaspoon salt
¼ Teaspoon pepper

Preheat oven to 450. In a small bowl, add milk, cayenne pepper, salt, and pepper. Mix to make a batter. Grind grissini in food processor until it's powder, then put the breadstick in a separate small bowl. Place rings in batter bowl and toss to coat fully. Let the rings sit in the batter for 2-3 minutes, then toss again. Dip each ring into the grissini powder by hand. Do it one at a time. Place on a cookie sheet lined with non-stick aluminum foil. Cook 6-7 minutes, then flip, cooking both sides.
Serving Size - 1 Vegetable, 1 Breadstick, 1 Milk

ROASTED GARLIC ASPARAGUS
2 cups asparagus
1-2 cloves minced garlic
¼ Teaspoon oregano
Black pepper (to taste)

Preheat oven to 400. Trim asparagus. Spread the spears on a sheet of non-stick aluminum foil. Add the seasonings. Wrap all ends of the foil up tightly to make a sealed 'pocket'. Roast 15-20 minutes
Serving Size - 1 Vegetable

CUCUMBER DILL SALAD
2 cups thinly sliced cucumbers
1 Tablespoon vinegar (to taste)
1 Teaspoon dill
½ Teaspoon Zsweet (as needed)
Black pepper

Combine all ingredients except cucumber & mix well. Toss in cucumbers. Cover & refrigerate. This tastes best if you wait at least one hour before serving.
Serving Size - 1 Vegetable

TANGY CRUNCHY CABBAGE
2 cups shredded cabbage
1/8 cup water
¼ cup apple cider vinegar
Salt and pepper to taste

Place all ingredients in a frying pan. Stir constantly until cabbage is at your desired consistency.

Serving Size - 1 Vegetable

CUCUMBER WITH MINT SALAD

2 cups cucumber - sliced or diced

1 Tablespoon vinegar (vary to taste - as I usually add about 3 Tablespoons)

1 Teaspoon black pepper

1 Teaspoon minced garlic

1 Teaspoon dried mint

Toss & mix all ingredients. Cover. Refrigerate for at least 1 hour. Toss before serving.

Serving Size - 1 Vegetable

LEMON GINGER ASPARAGUS

Asparagus (allowed amount)

½ cup water

½ Tablespoon fresh minced ginger root

3 cloves minced garlic

Lemon zest

Black pepper

Preheat pan over medium heat. Snap off 'woody' ends of asparagus spears & discard. Snap spears into 2-3 pieces. Add garlic & ginger to the pan and cook for 2-3 minutes. Add asparagus & water. Bring to a boil for 5 minutes. Remove asparagus and top with lemon rind & pepper, then serve.

Serving Size - 1 Vegetable

Soups (11)

CINNAMON CURRY CHICKEN SOUP

100 grams cooked chicken breast - cubed
1 cup diced onion
2 cups water
3 cloves minced garlic
½ Teaspoon curry powder
¼ Teaspoon cinnamon
Salt and black pepper to taste

In saucepan, combine all ingredients. Bring to a boil. Reduce heat, cover and simmer for 45 minutes.
Serving Size - 1 Protein, 1 Vegetable

CHICKEN RADISH SOUP

Radishes (sliced or coarsely chopped - however you prefer)
100 grams cooked chicken breast - cubed
1-2 cloves minced garlic
2 cups water (vary liquid amount depending on amount of soup desired)
Salt to taste
Pepper to taste

Combine all ingredients in saucepan. Bring to a boil. Reduce heat and simmer 10-15 minutes. Serve immediately.
Serving Size - 1 Protein, 1 Vegetable

CREAM OF CHICKEN SOUP

100 grams cooked chicken breast
2 cups celery - chopped
1 - 2 cups water
3 cloves garlic
½ Teaspoon parsley
½ Teaspoon basil
Ground white pepper to taste
Salt (optional)

Preheat saucepan to medium-high heat. In food processor combine all ingredients and pulse until it reaches your desired consistency. Pour into saucepan and bring to a boil. Reduce heat to simmer, cover and heat 20-30 minutes.
Serving Size - 1 Protein, 1 Vegetable

LEMON CHICKEN SOUP

100 grams shredded or diced chicken breast
2 cups chopped spinach
2-3 cups water
Juice of 1 lemon
1 teaspoon of thyme
Sea salt to taste
Ground white pepper to taste

Preheat saucepan over medium heat. Combine all ingredients. Bring to a boil, then simmer for 20 minutes and serve.

Serving Size - 1 Protein, 1 Vegetable, 1 Lemon

FRENCH ONION SOUP

2 cups Chicken Bouillon Base (below)
1 whole sliced sweet onion

Combine boullion base along with the sliced onion. Place in a pan and cook over medium heat until onions are tender.
Serving Size - 1 Protein, 1 Vegetable

ITALIAN BEEF SOUP

100 grams ground London Broil or Round Roast
1 large or 2 small tomatoes
1-2 cups water (adjust to how 'soupy' you'd like it)
1 clove garlic
1/8 Teaspoon oregano
1/8 Teaspoon white pepper
1/8 Teaspoon Italian Seasoning
Sea salt to taste

Combine chopped tomato, minced garlic, spices and ground beef prepared on a George Forman grill (or fry and drain well). Saute until heated through.
Serving Size - 1 Protein, 1 Vegetable

HOT & SOUR SHRIMP SOUP

100 grams shrimp (may use chicken instead)
2 cups bok choy OR asparagus
2 cups water

1 Teaspoon sambal oelek
½ Teaspoon white pepper
¼ Teaspoon ginger
Crushed red pepper

In saucepan, combine water, ginger, sambal oelek and white pepper. Bring to a boil. Reduce heat, cover and simmer for 2-3 minutes. Add shrimp. Return to a boil. Add vegetable, cover, and simmer for 2-3 minutes. Sprinkle with crushed red pepper and serve.
Serving Size - 1 Protein, 1 Vegetable

YOURHCG.COM CHICKEN BROTH

6 - 100 gram pieces of chicken breast
8 cups water
¼ Teaspoon garlic powder
¼ Teaspoon poultry seasoning
¼ Teaspoon black pepper
1 ½ Teaspoon sea salt

Combine ingredients in soup pot and cook until chicken is done. Remove chicken and refrigerate or freeze to use at a later time (I like to save it to put on salads). Also freeze bouillon base for future recipes. Put 2 cups in a medium size container to make soups or 4 tablespoons in a small container to sauté.
Serving Size - 1 Protein

CHICKEN (FORGO THE) TORTILLA SOUP

3 medium tomatoes
1 Tablespoon minced garlic
1 Tablespoon cumin

¼ teaspoon red pepper
Pinch of sea salt
½ Teaspoon black pepper
2 Tablespoons liquid aminos
½ cup water
4 Tablespoons fresh cilantro
100 grams cooked/shredded chicken breast
1 Melba toast or Grissini breadstick

Preheat pot over medium-high heat. Blanch 3 tomatoes in boiling water, drain and drench in cold water, peel skins and crush in the pot with your fingers or fork. Add minced garlic, cumin, chili powder, cayenne, red pepper, salt and black pepper. Continue to crush the tomatoes to your desired consistency with a fork. Add 1-2 tbsp liquid aminos (you don't have to be precise...I just throw a bit in for good measure). Add 1/4-1/2 cup water. Add 2 of the 4 tablespoons of fresh chopped cilantro. Bring to low boil. Reduce heat to a simmer and add chicken. Simmer for 10 minutes. Stir in last bit of cilantro before serving. Serve with your Grissini breadstick on the side or break into 1" pieces on top like traditional tortilla soup.
Serving Size - 1 Protein, 1 Vegetable, 1 Breadstick

HOT & SPICY WHITE CHILI

100 grams cooked chicken breast, shredded
1 cup diced onion or 1 large tomato
1-4 cups water (depending on how soupy you want it)
2 cloves minced garlic
½ Teaspoon chili powder
1/8 Teaspoon garlic powder
½ Teaspoon cumin

¼ Teaspoon oregano
¼ Teaspoon red pepper flakes
1/8 Teaspoon ground cloves
3 -4 shakes sugar free hot sauce to taste

Preheat pot over medium-high heat. Add all ingredients except for Tabasco/hot sauce. Bring to a boil then reduce heat to simmer, cover, & cook 30 minutes Add Tabasco or hot sauce right before serving.
TIP: This is also great fixed in a small crock pot. Toss everything in and put it on while you're out and come back to great tasting dinner! If using the crock pot, you can use cut up uncooked chicken.
Serving Size - 1 Protein, 1 Vegetable

YOURHCG.COM STEW
100 grams chopped London Broil or Round Roast
¼ Teaspoon salt
1/8 Teaspoon pepper
1/8 Teaspoon thyme
1/8 Teaspoon marjoram
1/8 Teaspoon rosemary
1/8 Teaspoon basil
1/8 Teaspoon sage
1 chopped tomato
2 Tablespoons apple cider vinegar

Sauté tomato in apple cider vinegar for about 5-7 minutes. Add meat and brown. Add the rest of the spices along with 1cup water. Bring to a boil, then reduce heat and simmer for 45 minutes.
Serving Size - 1 Protein, 1 Vegetable

Salads (9)

CUCUMBER SALAD

2 cups thinly sliced cucumber
1 Tablespoon vinegar (to taste)
1 Teaspoon dill
Black pepper (to taste)

Combine all ingredients except cucumber. Mix well. Toss in the cucumbers. Cover & refrigerate for at least 1 hour.
Serving Size - 1 Vegetable

BIZ'S THAI CUCUMBER BEEF SALAD

100 grams London broil or round roast
1 Teaspoon sambal oelek or red pepper flakes
2-3 cloves minced garlic
¼ Teaspoon ground white pepper
2-3 Tablespoons water
2 cups cucumber
Juice of 1/2 lemon
Chopped cilantro

Peel, seed, and slice cucumber. In small dish, combine cucumber, juice of 1/2 lemon, and chopped cilantro. Toss. Cover & refrigerate to marinate while preparing the rest of the dish. Preheat pan over medium-high heat. Slice steak into very thin slices. In small bowl, place steak, sambal oelek, garlic, and white pepper. Be sure to coat steak well. Place steak in pan with water. Stir fry for 2-5 minutes depending on how you like your steak cooked. Serve immediately while hot over cold cucumbers.
Serving Size - 1 Protein, 1 Vegetable, ½ Lemon

CUCUMBER SHRIMP SALAD

1 cup diced cucumber

100 grams cooked shrimp, diced

White vinegar (to taste)

½ Lemon (to taste)

Sugar free hot sauce (to taste)

Place all the ingredients in a bowl and toss.

Serving Size - 1 Protein, 1 Cucumber, ½ Lemon

SPICY CRAB CUCUMBER SALAD

100 grams crab - shredded

2 cups cucumber - peeled, seeded, and julienned

1 Tablespoon amino acids

½ - 1 Tablespoon dry mustard

½ - 1 Teaspoon wasabi powder

Grissini breadstick - coarsely ground

Combine liquid aminos, dry mustard and wasabi powder. Stir. Add remaining ingredients, toss & serve.

Serving Size - 1 Protein, 1 Vegetable, 1 Breadstick

SHRIMP SALAD WITH VINAIGRETTE DRESSING

2 cups raw spinach
100 grams grilled shrimp
Dash of garlic salt
Vinaigrette Dressing (found in "sauces" section)
1 piece Melba toast or 1 Grissini Breadstick

Grill shrimp and dash with garlic salt. Arrange spinach on plate and add shrimp. Spray or spoon on Vinaigrette Dressing. Serve with Melba toast or Grissini breadstick.
Serving Size - 1 Protein, 1 Vegetable, 1 Breadstick

CRUNCHY ASIAN SALAD

2 cups romaine lettuce or spinach
1 chopped orange
100 grams chicken breast
¼ Teaspoon Chinese 5 spice
1/8 Teaspoon garlic salt
1 packet Stevia
1 piece of Melba Toast
Citrus Dressing (recipe in "sauces" section)

Cook and chop chicken. Toss lettuce, orange, and chicken with Chinese Five Spice, garlic salt and Stevia. Break Melba toast into small pieces, like croutons. Spray or spoon on Citrus Dressing.
Serving Size - 1 Protein, 1 Vegetable, 1 Fruit, 1 Melba Toast

YOURHCG.COM TACO SALAD

2 cups romaine lettuce
100 grams London Broil or Round Roast (can also use chicken breast)
¼ cup water
¼ Teaspoon garlic powder
¼ Teaspoon chili powder
¼ Teaspoon cayenne
1 Onion flavored Melba Toasts
HCG Vinaigrette Dressing (removed)

Brown beef or chicken with seasonings. Drain well!
Top lettuce with ground beef mixture. Sprinkle with ground Melba toast.
Serving Size - 1 Protein, 1 Vegetable, 1 Melba toast

YOURHCG.COM CHOPPED CHICKEN SALAD

100 grams chicken breast - cut into small chunks
½ cup water
2 cups cabbage - chopped
Pepper to taste
Salt to taste
1 Apple - chopped into small chunks
1 Melba toast or Grissini breadstick

Warm up chicken along with water. You can boil the chicken and use the water that's left over as broth for this same meal. Pour chicken over bed of cabbage and let the cabbage absorb the water. Sprinkle with salt and pepper. Add apple chunks and mix the salad together. You may use one of the HCG friendly dressings with this salad as well, if the broth doesn't work for you.

Serving Size - 1 Protein, 1 Vegetable, 1 Fruit, 1 Breadstick

LEMON CHICKEN SALAD

2 cups raw spinach or romaine lettuce
½ cup chopped apple
100 grams chicken breast (Use Lemon Rosemary Chicken recipe)
Your favorite HCG dressing

Cook and chop chicken. Arrange spinach or lettuce on plate, sprinkle with chopped apple and chopped chicken. Spray or spoon on dressing.
Serving Size - 1 Protein, 1 Vegetable, 1 Fruit, ½ Lemon

Protein Shake Recipes (4)

**Protein shakes were not on the original protocol, use at your own risk.

VANILLA SHAKE

1 cup water
1 scoop MRM 100% Natural Whey protein powder - vanilla
Blend and enjoy. May also add Vanilla Creme Stevia drops for a more vanilla flavor OR add your favorite flavored Stevia drops.
Serving Size - 1 Protein

STRAWBERRY SHAKE

1 cup water
1 scoop MRM 100% Natural Whey protein powder - vanilla
One cup of frozen strawberries

Blend and enjoy.
Serving Size - 1 Protein, 1 Fruit

ORANGE VANILLA SHAKE

1 cup water
1 scoop MRM 100% Natural Whey protein powder - vanilla
1 orange

Blend and enjoy.
Serving Size - 1 Protein, 1 Fruit

CHOCOLATE SHAKE

1 cup water
1 scoop MRM 100% Natural Whey protein powder - Dutch chocolate
2 Tablespoon defatted cocoa (found at health food stores)

Blend and enjoy. May also add flavored Stevia drops for a more "chocolate" taste.
Serving Size - 1 Protein

Desserts and Fruits (9)

CINNAMON APPLESAUCE

5 apples
The juice of ½ lemon
½ cup water
1 packet Stevia
½ Teaspoon cinnamon

Peel, core and chop apples. Cook apples and water in a crock pot on low for 2 hours. When cooled, puree apples in blender while adding Stevia and cinnamon. Divide into 5 equal portions.
Serving Size - 1 Fruit, ½ Lemon

CINNAMON SPICED GRAPEFRUIT

1/2 grapefruit
Cinnamon
1-2 packets Stevia
2 Tablespoons water

Using a serrated edge knife, cut grapefruit in half as normally would and place on a microwave safe plate. Cut around center core, rind, and partitions. Place cinnamon, Stevia and water in a bowl to make a paste. Pour sauce over grapefruit. Heat in microwave on high for 2 minutes.
Serving Size - 1 Fruit

YOURHCG.COM FRIENDLY APPLE COBBLER

1 sliced apple
1/8 Teaspoon cinnamon
1 packet Stevia
1 Tablespoon milk

Toss the above ingredients and arrange on a microwave safe plate.

Topping:
1 Melba Toast
Cinnamon
¼ packet Stevia

Sprinkle apples with crumbled Melba Toast rounds, cinnamon and 1/4 packet Stevia. Heat in microwave for 2 minutes.
Serving Size - 1 Fruit, 1 Milk, 1 Melba Toast

STRAWBERRY SORBET

One cup of strawberries
Juice of 1 lemon
Stevia (as needed)
Water (if needed)

Freeze fresh strawberries about 1 hour. Blend fresh strawberries, lemon juice & Stevia in blender until very well blended. You can serve immediately or place in freezer to allow it to firm up even further.
Serving Size - 1 Fruit, 1 Lemon

BROILED CINNAMON GRAPEFRUIT

1/2 grapefruit
cinnamon to taste (optional)
Zsweet (as needed)

Take a knife around the inside peel of the grapefruit so that it cuts out the grapefruit from the peel. Separate the sections and place in a bowl. Sprinkle with Zsweet and cinnamon. Toss, place back into grapefruit peel. Broil for about 3-5 minutes until carmelized.
Serving Size - 1 Fruit

APPLESAUCE
1 apple
3 Tablespoons water
Cinnamon (optional)

Peel, core, and dice apple. Place diced apple in mini-crockpot and add water. Add cinnamon. Cook at least two hours. When finished, mash with spoon or fork, or place in blender to reach desired consistency. Serve warm or refrigerate and serve cold.
Serving Size - 1 Fruit

WARM CINNAMON APPLE
1 apple
Cinnamon to taste
Stevia to taste

Cut one apple in half and sprinkle enough cinnamon on the apple to completely cover the exposed tops. Place them on a plate and microwave for 2-3 minutes.
Serving Size - 1 Fruit

VANILLA STRAWBERRY DESSERT

Handful of strawberries
5 drops Vanilla Crème Stevia
8-10 drops Chocolate or Chocolate Raspberry Stevia
1 Tablespoon milk

Mix milk, Vanilla Crème Stevia, and Chocolate Stevia in a bowl. Mix in sliced strawberries and enjoy.
Serving Size - 1 Fruit, 1 Milk

YourHCG.com Friendly 'Pie'

1 apple OR cup of strawberries
Sprinkle of cinnamon
Few drops of Vanilla Creme Stevia

Cut apples or strawberries into slices. Place in a saucepan on medium heat and sprinkle with cinnamon. Add a little water to the pan and simmer until fruit is soft. Then add a few drops of Vanilla Creme Stevia.
Serving Size - 1 Fruit

YOURHCG.COM BASIC SEASONING

**** This seasoning is great for beef, chicken and seafood.**

1 Tablespoon garlic powder

2 Tablespoons dried sage leaves, crumbled

2 Tablespoons dried parsley leaves

2 Tablespoons dried thyme leaves

2 Tablespoons rosemary

2 Tablespoons white pepper

Combine all of the ingredients in a bowl. Put in container with a tight fitting lid and store away from heat and light. Shake or stir to re-blend before each use.

INDIAN CURRY SEASONING

1 Tablespoon tumeric

1 Tablespoon coriander

2 Teaspoons paprika

1 Teaspoon pepper

1 Teaspoon cumin

1 Teaspoon ginger

½ Teaspoon cloves

½ Teaspoon celery seed

½ Teaspoon cayenne

Mix and store in an airtight container.

SEAFOOD SEASONING

1 Tablespoon ground bay leaves
2 ½ Teaspoons celery seed
1 ½ Teaspoons dry mustard
1 ½ Teaspoons black pepper
¾ Teaspoon ground nutmeg
½ Teaspoon ground cloves
½ Teaspoon ground ginger
½ Teaspoon paprika
½ Teaspoon red pepper
¼ Teaspoon ground cardamom
¼ Teaspoon ground mace

Mix all ingredients and store in an airtight container.

MOCK SHAKE N BAKE

¼ Teaspoon coriander
¼ Teaspoon thyme
¼ Teaspoon red pepper flakes
1/8 Teaspoon oregano
1/8 Teaspoon paprika
1/8 Teaspoon black pepper
1/8 Teaspoon salt

Place all ingredients in a food processor or coffee grinder. Grind to a powder. Store in an air tight container.

MARINARA SAUCE

1 large tomato
Water
1 Teaspoon oregano
1 Teaspoon basil
2 Tablespoons parsley
1 clove garlic (fresh, minced)
1 Teaspoon salt
¼ Teaspoon pepper

Fill small saucepan with a few cups of water and bring to a boil. Score skin of tomato in a few places with a serrated knife. Blanch tomato in the boiling water for 1-2 minutes. Immediately transfer tomato to ice water to cool and discard boiling water. Remove skin of tomato and discard skin. Preheat small non-stick saucepan over MED-HI heat If you want chunky sauce, crush tomato with your hand in a sauce pan. If you prefer smoother sauce, puree tomato in blender then add to the pan. Add garlic, salt & pepper Bring to a low boil, then immediately reduce heat to low, cover & simmer for 15 minutes, stirring often to keep from sticking. Turn heat up to MED. Add parsley, oregano, more garlic and basil. Cook 5-10 minutes stirring constantly. While cooking, start adding water 1Tablespoon at a time until it reaches your desired consistency.
Serving Size - 1 Vegetable

CARIBBEAN CHICKEN RUB

1 Tablespoon parsley
1 Teaspoon cumin
1 Teaspoon chili powder
½ Teaspoon black pepper
½ Teaspoon allspice
¼ Teaspoon cinnamon

This amount makes enough for 2 servings of chicken (possibly even more depending on how much seasoning you like) so you can shake both of them up in the zip lock, cook both, and then refrigerate the extra chicken.

BBQ RUB

2 Tablespoons paprika
1 Tablespoon granulated sugar substitute
1 Tablespoon ground cumin
1 Tablespoon black pepper
1 Tablespoon chili powder

Mix; store in air-tight container/zip lock bag.

CAJUN SEASONING

1 Tablespoon chili powder
1 Tablespoon Hungarian paprika
1 Teaspoon garlic powder
½ Teaspoon dried oregano
½ Teaspoon dried thyme
½ Teaspoon cayenne pepper
½ Teaspoon freshly ground pepper

Combine & store in airtight container.

GREEK SEASONING MIX

2 Teaspoons oregano
1 ½ Teaspoons garlic powder
1 Teaspoon salt
1 Teaspoon black pepper
1 Teaspoon parsley
1 Teaspoon basil
½ Teaspoon cinnamon
½ Teaspoon nutmeg
½ Teaspoon thyme

Grind spices in food processor or coffee grinder. Store in an airtight container.

EMERIL'S 'SOUTHWEST SPICE'

2 Tablespoons chili powder
1 Tablespoon dried oregano
2 Tablespoons paprika
1 Tablespoon ground coriander
1 Tablespoon garlic powder
1 Tablespoon salt
2 Teaspoons ground cumin
1 Teaspoon black pepper
1 Teaspoon cayenne pepper
1 Teaspoon ground red pepper

Combine all ingredients thoroughly and store in an airtight container.

APPLE CIDER VINEGAR DRESSING

2/3 cup water
1/3 cup Apple Cider Vinegar
Stevia powder of liquid drops to taste
Salt and pepper to taste

Mix the water and Apple Cider Vinegar together, stir or shake, and then add Stevia drops or powder to taste into the mixture. Finally, pour over your lettuce.

ASIAN CITRUS DRESSING

¼ cup apple cider vinegar
1 cup water
1 Tablespoon fresh lemon juice
15 drops Clear Stevia
10 drops Apricot Nectar flavored Stevia
1 packet Stevia
¼ Teaspoon Chinese Style Five Spice (optional)
¼ Teaspoon garlic salt (optional)
Dash of curry seasoning
Dash of cumin

Combine ingredients, pour into jar and refrigerate.

VINAIGRETTE DRESSING

¼ apple cider vinegar
1 cup water
Ground pepper to taste
20 drops Clear Stevia
3 packets Stevia

Combine ingredients, pour into jar and refrigerate.

Beverages (8)

Carbonated water is not allowed while on the low calorie diet.

ROOT BEER
8 oz carbonated water
15 drops Root Beer Stevia

Mix in a glass over ice and enjoy.

CITRUS BURST
8 oz. carbonated water
10 drops Lemon Drop Stevia
5 drops Apricot Nectar Stevia

Mix in a glass over ice and enjoy

GRAPE SODA
8 oz. carbonated water
10 drops Grape Stevia

Mix in a glass over ice and enjoy

MOCK 7-UP
8 oz carbonated water
10 drops Valencia Orange Stevia

Mix in a glass over ice and enjoy

ROOT BEER CREME

8 oz. carbonated water
13 drops Root Beer Stevia
3 drops Vanilla Creme Stevia

Mix in a glass over ice and enjoy

ORANGE SODA

8 ounces carbonated water
15 drops Valencia Orange Stevia

Mix in a glass over ice and enjoy

MOCK FRESCA

8 ounces carbonated water
10 drops Lemon Drop Stevia

Mix in a glass over ice and enjoy

STRAWBERRY ORANGE SMOOTHIE

¾ cup crushed ice
1 orange
1 cup fresh or partially defrosted strawberries
5 drops Clear Stevia
5 drops Valencia Orange Stevia
5 drops Vanilla Creme Stevia

Mix in a blender and serve in a tall glass. You can garnish with a lemon, lime an orange wedge.

SHRIMP CEVICHE

1 to 2 pounds shrimp, peeled and deveined, tail-on or off
2 large lemons, freshly squeezed
2-3 large limes, freshly squeezed
1 Tablespoon fresh garlic, minced
1 mild to medium pepper, ribs and seeds removed, finely chopped
1 red onion, finely chopped
1-3 tablespoons Tabasco or hot sauce
4 large tomatoes,
2 cucumbers, peeled and diced into 1/2 inch pieces fresh
½ cup each of freshly chopped cilantro and parsley
Sea salt and fresh ground black pepper to taste

Thaw shrimp if frozen. If using raw shrimp, bring a pot of water to boil and cook the shrimp for a minute or two until it turns opaque white and reddish—do not overcook the shrimp as it will be too rubbery in texture. Rinse shrimp under cold water. Combine juices of lemons and limes in a large bowl (not metal) or large Ziploc baggie and add shrimp. Cover bowl or zip baggie and refrigerate for 30 minutes to marinade. Large shrimp could be cut into smaller chunks (remove tails if doing this) to speed up marinade time. Add to shrimp the Tabasco, garlic, onion and pepper and toss/mix evenly. Return to refrigerator for maybe another 30 minutes to let the flavors infuse the shrimp. Before serving, toss in bowl the marinated shrimp mixture, cilantro, parsley, tomatoes and cucumbers and if needed, add sea salt and black pepper to taste.

Chicken (2)

SALSA CHICKEN

100 grams chicken breast
Salsa with no added sugars or preservatives

Place chicken in crockpot with salsa. Cook for 6 hours.

MEXICAN CHICKEN LETTUCE WRAPS

3.5 ounces of chopped chicken breast
¼ cup organic chicken broth
¼ cup finely diced white onion
1 garlic clove pressed
Fresh herbs to taste (cilantro, oregano, parsley)
Dried spices to taste (cumin, chili powder, salt, pepper)
2 large butter leaf lettuce leaves (for taco shells)

In a small pan, sauté onions, garlic and spices (not herbs) in the chicken broth. When onions are starting to caramelize, add chicken. Cook completely. Spoon out mixture into large butter leaves and garnish with fresh herbs. Add fresh organic salsa if desired.

Beef (2)

GROUND BEEF TACOS

1 pound Extra Lean Ground Beef
½ Teaspoon cumin
¼ Teaspoon salt
¼ Teaspoon black pepper
¼ Teaspoon chili pepper
¼ Teaspoon onion powder
¼ Teaspoon garlic powder
1 Roma tomato, diced
1 avocado, sliced
½ red onion, diced
Romaine Lettuce, complete leaves

Brown beef in a frying pot. Mix the cumin, black pepper, chili pepper, onion salt, and garlic powder in a bowl. Add seasonings to the ground beef to your taste. Add a dash of regular salt if needed. Cut up Roma tomato, slice up avocado and dice some red onion and set aside. Take leaves of romaine lettuce. Add some meat and the tomatoes, onion and avocado (and cheese if preferred) and eat it like a taco.

FAJITAS

1 ½ pounds chicken or beef
1 medium onion, sliced
1 green bell pepper, sliced
2 cups mushrooms, sliced
1 clove garlic, minced
1 cup low sodium Beef Broth
¼ Teaspoon paprika, pepper, salt and cayenne

In a cast iron skillet, grill chicken or beef, add garlic, onions, and bell pepper. Add paprika, cracked pepper, salt and cayenne. Add broth and cover. Cook for 20 minutes over medium heat. Serve with no added sugar salsa and sour cream.

Vegetables (4)

FRITTATA

1 pound of vegetables (broccoli, spinach, etc.)
½ onion, diced
Handful of sliced mushrooms
8 Eggs
1 cup Milk
3 ounces parmesan cheese
2 cups Mozzarella
Salt, pepper and basil to taste

Preheat oven to 350 degrees. Sauté onions and mushrooms in some butter until they are tender. While those are cooking, beat eggs in a bowl, then add a cup of milk to it and about 3 ounces of parmesan cheese along with some salt/pepper and some basil. After the veggies are steamed and sautéed then I spray a 13 x 9 baking dish with Olive Oil Pam and put the veggies on the bottom making it as even as possible. Pour the egg, cheese, spics, and milk mixture over veggies. Then sprinkle 2 handfuls of mozzarella cheese over the top. Bake, uncovered for about 20 minutes. The eggs should NOT be all the way set. Then switch the oven over to BROIL and watch closely until the cheese starts to bubble. Remove and cool and cut into serving squares. Put them in individual sandwich bags and freeze.

STEAMED KALE

1 bunch of fresh kale, chopped
¼ onion, chopped
2 garlic cloves, minced
1 cup water
Braggs liquid aminos
Salt and Pepper to taste

Place the onion, garlic, kale, salt, pepper and water in large pan. Bring to a boil. Cover and simmer for about 30 minutes (until kale is tender). Sprinkle with liquid aminos.

FAUX MASHED POTATOES

1 pound cauliflower
1 Tablespoon water
1 Tablespoon butter
1-2 Tablespoons heavy cream
Salt and pepper

Chop the cauliflower into small pieces and place in large covered casserole dish. Add water and microwave on high for 5 minutes. Stir and cook another 5 minutes. Let stand covered 5 more minutes, then drain. Place in a food processor or blender with butter and heavy cream. Process until smooth and creamy, scraping down the sides of the processor occasionally. Season with salt and pepper.

ROASTED VEGETABLES

1 medium purple onion

1 pound asparagus
1 pound mushrooms, any variety
1 yellow bell pepper
1 orange bell pepper
2 medium tomatoes, seeded
1 zucchini
1 yellow squash
Olive oil
Salt and pepper

Preheat oven to 350 degrees. Wash and chop veggies into bite size, pieces. Add all veggies to a bowl. Drizzle with olive oil and salt/pepper. Use a spatula to thoroughly coat veggies. Spread veggies into a shallow baking dish. Bake uncovered until veggies are crunchy tender.

Soups (3)

VEGETARIAN CHOWDER

1 medium onion, chopped
3-4 celery stalks, chopped
1/3 of a green pepper, chopped
2 cups cauliflower, chopped
3 cups of broccoli, chopped
¼ head of green cabbage, chopped
10 Crimini mushrooms, chopped
2- 3 cloves of garlic
2 Tablespoons butter
2 Tablespoons flour
1 quart half and half milk
1 quart of no sodium chicken stock
2 ½ cups shredded medium cheddar

Sauté onion, celery and green pepper in a frying pan. Once softened, add 2-3 cloves of garlic. Cook until garlic is incorporated. Move to your main pot. In a steamer, steam cauliflower, broccoli, green cabbage and mushrooms together for 10 minutes. Puree half of the steamed veggies. Mix them with the other veggie mix in the main pot. In a frying pan add 2 Tablespoons of butter and flour. Heat through then add ¾ quart of half & half, salt and pepper to make a rue. Stir until smooth then add 1 ½ cups of shredded cheese and 1 ½ cups no sodium chicken stock. Add to taste garlic powder and onion powder. Then add 1 teaspoon pepper, ½ teaspoon seasoning salt and sea salt. Stir until smooth and pour over veggies in the main pot. Simmer over medium until desired consistency. Add remaining milk or additional chicken stock to thin.

ALBONDIGAS SOUP

1 serving meatballs
2-3 cups beef or chicken broth
100 - 200grams bok choy, onion or cabbage
Fresh chopped cilantro
Seasonings to taste

In saucepan, bring broth to a boil. Feel free to add any seasonings you like to taste (oregano, basil, pepper, garlic, etc.). I'll usually add in some hot sauce or Tabasco. Add cooked meatballs and veggie choice. Cover & simmer 20-30 minutes or until vegetables reach desired tenderness. Top with fresh chopped cilantro. Serve.

LEFTOVER TURKEY SOUP

2 c. water or no sodium added chicken broth
10-12 oz turkey breast
1 large onion, chopped
3 celery sticks, shopped
2 cups tomatoes, chopped
2 Tablespoons minced garlic
½ pkg frozen chopped spinach, thawed and drained
1 Tablespoon chopped parsley
1/8 Teaspoon marjoram
1 bay leaf
1/8 teaspoon poultry seasoning
1/8 teaspoon thyme

Combine all ingredients except parsley (if using fresh) and spinach in crock pot. Cook all day on low heat. 1 hour before serving, add spinach and fresh parsley. Salt and pepper to taste.

Salads (1)

YOURHCG.COM CHEF SALAD

Handful of assorted greens
1 tomato, chopped
½ cucumber, sliced and seeded
¼ cup ham
¼ cup turkey
2 hard boiled eggs
Favorite YourHCG.com vinaigrette

Place all of the ingredients and enjoy.

'Breads' (5)

OOPSIE ROLLS

3 large eggs
Dash of salt
Pinch of cream of tartar
3 ounces cream cheese (Do not soften)

Preheat oven to 300. Separate the eggs. Add salt and cream cheese to the yolks. Use a mixer to combine the ingredients together. In a separate bowl, whip egg whites and cream of tartar until stiff (if you're using the same mixer, mix the whites first and then the yolk mixture). Using a spatula, gradually fold the egg yolk mixture into the white mixture, being careful not to break down the whites. Spray a cookie sheet with non-stick spray and spoon the mixture onto the sheet, making 6 mounds. Flatten each mound slightly. Bake on parchment paper about 30 minutes (You want them slightly softer, not crumbly). Let cool on the sheet for a few minutes, and then remove to a rack and allow them to cool. Store them in a bread sack or a sandwich bag.

PIZZA CRUST

2 cups mozzarella cheese
2 large eggs
2 Tablespoons flax seed meal
2 Tablespoons coconut flour
1/2 Teaspoon baking soda

Mix all together. If you have a pizza stone, it's good to use but if you don't just use a cookie sheet. Put the dough between two sheets of parchment paper and roll really thin Make sure there are no holes, about a 1/4" thickness. Remove the top sheet and bake at 350 for 15 minutes. Place the top sheet back on, flip and bake about 5-10 minutes and then add your toppings. Bake or broil until bubbly.

PO' CAKES

2 eggs
7 Tablespoons almond flour
Pinch of salt

Heat skillet with oil. Mix eggs, flour and salt in a bowl until well blended. Drop by large spoonfuls and smooth out a bit. Cook on each side about 1-2 minutes until brown and a bit crunchy. Top with cream cheese or sugar free preserves of your choice.

VARIATION OF PO' CAKES

2 eggs
1/3 cup almond meal
Splash of milk
Pinch of salt
1 packet Stevia

Preheat skillet with coconut oil. Mix eggs, almond meal, milk, salt and Stevia in a bowl until well blended. In a frying pan or on a skillet, drop mixture making about 3 inch circles. Cook until light brown on one side, then flip until cooked all the way through.

CAULIFLOWER PIZZA CRUST

1 cup cauliflower, cooked
1 egg
1 cup mozzarella cheese
½ teaspoon fennel
1 Teaspoon oregano
2 Teaspoons parsley
Pizza or Alfredo sauce
Toppings (make sure meats are cooked)
Mozzarella cheese

Preheat oven to 450 degrees. Spray a cookie sheet with non-stick spray. In a medium bowl, combine cauliflower, egg and mozzarella. Press evenly on the pan. Sprinkle evenly with fennel, oregano and parsley. Bake at 450 degrees for 12-15 minutes (15-20 minutes if you double the recipe). Remove the pan from the oven. To the crust, add sauce, then toppings and cheese. Place under a broiler at high heat just until cheese is melted.

CHEESCAKE

16 ounces cream cheese
12 packets Stevia
3 large eggs
3 Tablespoons fresh lemon juice
1 ½ Teaspoons vanilla extract - sugar free
¼ Teaspoon salt
3 cups sour cream

Preheat the oven to 350 F. In a large mixing bowl, beat the cream cheese and sweetener until very smooth, about 3 minutes. Add the eggs, one at a time, beating well after each addition. Add the lemon juice, vanilla and salt. Beat in the sour cream until just blended. Grease an 8-inch Springform pan with 2 1/2 inch sides and line the bottom with greased parchment or wax paper. Wrap the outside of the pan with a double layer of heavy duty foil to prevent seepage. Pour the batter into the pan. Set the pan in a large roasting pan and surround with 1 inch of very hot water. Bake for 45 minutes. Turn off the oven without opening the door and let the cake cool for 1 hour. Remove to a rack and cool to room temperature, about 1 hour. Cover with plastic wrap and refrigerate overnight. Un-mold the cake onto a plate.

APPLES WITH CREAMY STRAWBERRY SAUCE

1/2 Jonathon apple

3-5 small to medium strawberries

2 Tablespoons milk

3 drops Vanilla Creme Stevia

Slice apple and arrange on a plate. Mash the strawberries with a fork and add Vanilla Creme Stevia and milk to make a sauce. Pour over the apple slices.

MUG CAKE

4 Tablespoons almond flour

4 Tablespoons Stevia

2 Tablespoons Cocoa Powder (may also use sugar free peanut butter or cinnamon)

1 egg

3 Tablespoons milk

3 Tablespoons oil

Splash of vanilla extract (sugar free)

Mix dry ingredients in a coffee mug, add egg and blend. Add milk, oil, vanilla and blend. Microwave for three minutes. Let cool and place on plate.

GLUTEN FREE ALMOND CREPES

1 1/2 cup water
6 eggs
1 1/2 cups almond flour
2-3 Tablespoons Coconut Flour
1/2 Teaspoon Sea Salt
Allow batter to rest for 30 minutes.

Preheat non-stick 10" skillet and coat with oil, spray, or butter. In a large bowl, beat together 1 ½ cups water, 6 eggs, 1 ½ cups almond flour, 2-3 Tablespoons coconut flour and ½ teaspoon salt. Mix batter for a few seconds before making each crepe as it separates very quickly. Pour about 3 Tablespoons of batter into the pan, and lift the pan and tip it around to distribute evenly. Cook on medium heat until light brown on the bottom. Do not try to remove too soon because they will collapse and be mushy. Gently slip a spatula under the crepe and flip. When done, turn out onto a clean kitchen towel to cool; afterward they can be stacked and won't stick to each other. I wrap them up in the same towel I cooled them on to absorb any subsequent moisture, lay them on a strong paper plate so they don't bend while storing and then put it all in a sandwich bag in the fridge.

SMOKY BBQ SAUCE
2 Tablespoons sugar free tomato sauce
2-3 Tablespoons water
½ Teaspoon dehydrated minced onion
½ Teaspoon apple cider vinegar
¼ Teaspoon sugar free Liquid Smoke
¼ Teaspoon paprika
¼ Teaspoon chili powder
1/8 Teaspoon cinnamon
1/8 Teaspoon cloves
¼ - ½ Teaspoon Stevia (if needed)
Salt/pepper to taste

In small non-stick saucepan, combine all ingredients and bring to boil. Reduce heat and simmer for 20 minutes. Makes enough for 1-2 servings.

EASY COCKTAIL SAUCE
½ cup sugar free catsup
1 Tablespoon Horseradish (drained)
1 Teaspoon Lemon juice
1 Tablespoon Tomato paste

Mix in a bowl and place in refrigerator.

BARBEQUE SAUCE

3 ounces tomato paste
¼ cup apple cider vinegar
3 Tablespoons lemon juice
1 Tablespoon hot sauce
1 Tablespoon minced onion
3 cloves garlic, crushed and minced
¼ Teaspoon chili powder
Liquid smoke to taste (sugar free)
½ Teaspoon garlic powder and onion powder
1 Teaspoon chopped parsley
Stevia to taste (Dark chocolate liquid)
Cayenne pepper, salt and pepper to taste
Water as needed to achieve desired consistency

In a small saucepan, combine all ingredients. Mix well and bring to a boil. Reduce heat and simmer for at least 5 minutes adding a little water to achieve desired consistency and to make sure it doesn't burn. Use as a barbeque sauce for chicken or beef.

MAYO

1 Egg
2 Tablespoons Apple Cider Vinegar
2 Tablespoons Water
½ Teaspoon sea salt
1/8 Teaspoon each: pepper, onion powder and garlic powder
12-15 drops Liquid Stevia
1 Cup oil of choice

Mix egg, vinegar and water in blender, add spices and slowly add the oil while blender is running.

Plateau Breakers and Weight Loss Optimizers

If you hit a “plateau” in your weight loss in the HCG diet, here are some suggestions to help you get over it… (These tips can also help maximize your weight loss!)

Increase water intake to 2-3 quarts per day. You want to drink 1/2 your weight in water per day. So if you weigh 200lbs, you’ll drink 100oz of water per day.

Try adding a glass or 2 of green tea to your day.

Don’t eat 2 apples for the two fruits or cut down on the size of the apples.

American beef is fatty. Cut it down or out. Seafood and chicken are much better choices.

Check all condiments for any form of sugar.

If mixing vegetables, stop.

Try leaving out one or both bread sticks or Melba toast.

Try adding 2 Tablespoons of apple cider vinegar to your daily routine.

Grapefruit is a known fat burner; add a serving to your diet.

Taking potassium supplements can help you lose weight. Potassium helps release fluid from the cells. Always consult your physician before adding in any new supplements.

Make sure you are not drinking any "diet" drinks. Any form of sugar or "non-sugar" besides stevia will slow your weight loss.

Try not to eat anything from suppertime until lunch the next day. Studies have shown that people on the diet lose more by skipping breakfast. (Still drink fluids!)

Try cutting down the amount of coffee and mint you are consuming. They can decrease your body's response to homeopathic products.